The Simple Dash Diet Meals

enjoy these delicious recipes for your desserts

Candace Hickman

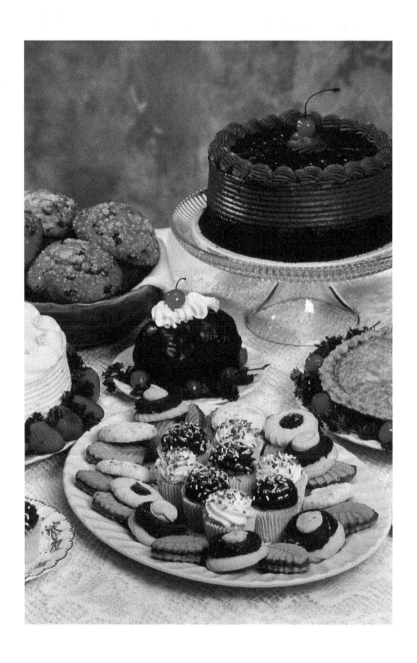

TABLE OF CONTENT

Coconut Pumpkin Cream

Preparation time: 2 hours

Cooking time: 0 minutes

Servings: 4

Ingredients:

- 2 cups coconut cream
- 1 cup pumpkin puree
- 3 tablespoons coconut sugar

Directions:

1. In a bowl, combine the cream with the pumpkin puree and the other ingredients, whisk well, divide into small bowls and keep in the fridge for 2 hours before serving.

Nutrition info per serving: 331calories, 3.4g protein, 20.6g carbohydrates, 28.8g fat, 4.4g fiber, 0g cholesterol, 21mg sodium, 442g potassium

Rhubarb and Figs Stew

Preparation time: 6 minutes

Cooking time: 14 minutes

Servings: 4

Ingredients:

- 2 tablespoons coconut oil, melted
- 1 cup rhubarb, roughly chopped
- 12 figs, halved
- ¼ cup of coconut sugar
- 1 cup of water

Directions:

1. Heat up a pan with the oil over medium heat, add the figs and the rest of the ingredients, toss, cook for 14 minutes, divide into small cups and serve cold.

Nutrition info per serving: 252calories, 2.2g protein, 49.8g carbohydrates, 7.4g fat, 6.1g fiber, 0g cholesterol, 9mg sodium, 476g potassium

Nutmeg Baked Bananas

Preparation time: 4 minutes

Cooking time: 15 minutes

Servings: 4

Ingredients:

- 4 bananas, peeled and halved

- 1 teaspoon nutmeg, ground

- 1 teaspoon cinnamon powder

- Juice of 1 lime

- 4 tablespoons coconut sugar

Directions:

1. Arrange the bananas in a baking pan, add the nutmeg and the other ingredients, bake at 350 degrees F for 15 minutes.
2. Divide the baked bananas between plates and serve.

Nutrition info per serving: 118calories, 1.4g protein, 29.6g carbohydrates, 0.6g fat, 3.2g fiber, 0g cholesterol, 2mg sodium, 450g potassium

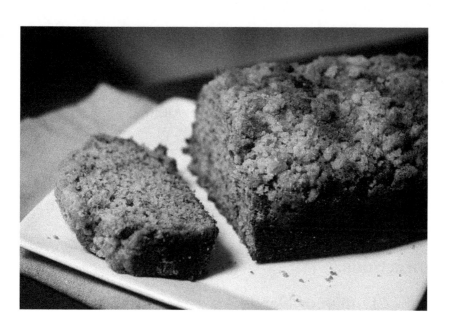

Coconut Avocado Smoothie

Preparation time: 5 minutes

Cooking time: 0 minutes

Servings: 2

Ingredients:

- 2 teaspoons cocoa powder
- 1 avocado, pitted, peeled and mashed
- 1 cup almond milk
- 1 cup coconut cream

Directions:

1. In your blender, combine the almond milk with the cream and the other ingredients, pulse well, divide into cups, and serve cold.

Nutrition info per serving: 515calories, 5.5g protein, 20.3g carbohydrates, 49.7g fat, 9.9g fiber, 0g cholesterol, 94mg sodium, 848g potassium

Banana and Avocado Bars

Preparation time: 30 minutes

Cooking time: 0 minutes

Servings: 4

Ingredients:

- 1 cup coconut oil, melted
- 2 bananas, peeled and chopped
- 1 avocado, peeled, pitted and mashed
- ½ cup of coconut sugar
- ¼ cup lime juice
- 1 teaspoon lemon zest, grated
- Cooking spray

Directions:

1. In your food processor, mix the bananas with the oil and the other ingredients except the cooking spray and pulse well.

2. Grease a pan with the cooking spray, pour and spread the banana mix, spread, keep in the fridge for 30 minutes, cut into bars, and serve.

Nutrition info per serving: 734calories, 1.8g protein, 46g carbohydrates, 64.6g fat, 5.2g fiber, 0g cholesterol, 13mg sodium, 503g potassium

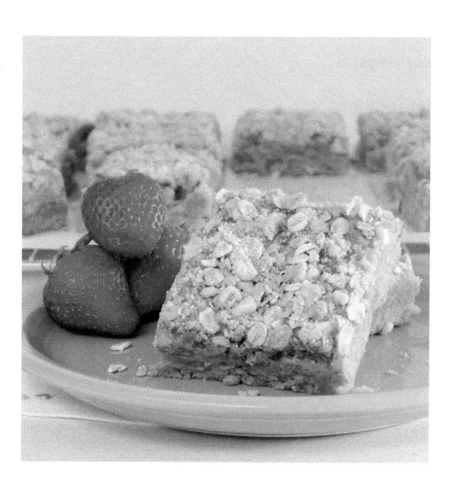

Vanilla Green Tea Bars

Preparation time: 10 minutes

Cooking time: 30 minutes

Servings: 8

Ingredients:

- 2 tablespoons green tea powder

- 2 cups coconut milk, heated

- ½ cup coconut oil, melted

- 2 cups of coconut sugar

- 4 eggs, whisked

- 2 teaspoons vanilla extract

- 3 cups almond flour

- 1 teaspoon baking soda

- 2 teaspoons baking powder

Directions:

1. In a bowl, combine the coconut milk with the green tea powder and the rest of the ingredients, stir well, pour into a square pan, spread, introduce in the oven, bake at 350 degrees F for 30 minutes, cool down, cut into bars and serve.

Nutrition info per serving: 544calories, 6.6g protein, 54g carbohydrates, 35.4g fat, 2.7g fiber, 82g cholesterol, 203mg sodium, 322g potassium

Coconut Walnut Cream

Preparation time: 2 hours

Cooking time: 0 minutes

Servings: 4

Ingredients:

- 2 cups almond milk
- ½ cup coconut cream
- ½ cup walnuts, chopped
- 3 tablespoons coconut sugar
- 1 teaspoon vanilla extract

Directions:

1. In a bowl, combine the almond milk with the cream and the other ingredients, whisk well, divide into cups and keep in the fridge for 2 hours before serving.

Nutrition info per serving: 409calories, 6.5g protein, 17.3g carbohydrates, 37.8g fat, 3.7g fiber, 0g cholesterol, 18mg sodium, 399g potassium

Almond Lemon Cake

Preparation time: 10 minutes

Cooking time: 35 minutes

Servings: 6

Ingredients:

- 2 cups whole wheat flour
- 1 teaspoon baking powder
- 2 tablespoons coconut oil, melted
- 1 egg, whisked
- 3 tablespoons coconut sugar
- 1 cup almond milk
- Zest of 1 lemon, grated
- Juice of 1 lemon

Directions:

1. In a bowl, combine the flour with the oil and the other ingredients, whisk well, transfer this to a cake pan and bake at 360 degrees F for 35 minutes.
2. Slice and serve cold.

Nutrition info per serving: 324calories, 6.2g protein, 42.3g carbohydrates, 15.3g fat, 2.1g fiber, 27g cholesterol, 35mg sodium, 252g potassium

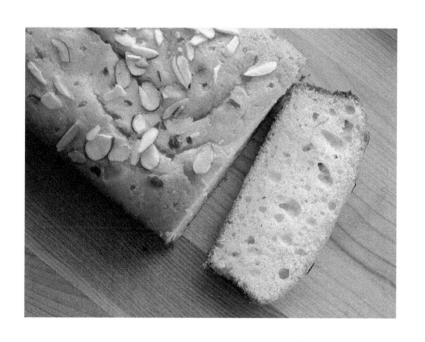

Cinnamon Bars

Preparation time: 10 minutes

Cooking time: 25 minutes

Servings: 6

Ingredients:

- 1 teaspoon cinnamon powder
- 2 cups almond flour
- 1 teaspoon baking powder
- ½ teaspoon nutmeg, ground
- 1 cup coconut oil, melted
- 1 cup of coconut sugar
- 1 egg, whisked
- 1 cup raisins

Directions:

1. In a bowl, combine the flour with the cinnamon and the other ingredients, stir well, spread on a lined baking sheet, introduce in the oven, bake at 380 degrees

F for 25 minutes, cut into bars and serve cold.

Nutrition info per serving: 579calories, 3.7g protein, 53.7g carbohydrates, 41.9g fat, 2g fiber, 27g cholesterol, 17mg sodium, 275g potassium

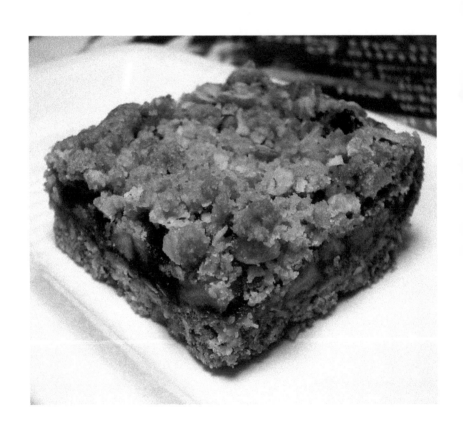

Nectarines Cocoa Squares

Preparation time: 10 minutes

Cooking time: 20 minutes

Servings: 4

Ingredients:

- 3 nectarines, pitted and chopped
- 1 tablespoon coconut sugar
- ½ teaspoon baking soda
- 1 cup almond flour
- 4 tablespoons coconut oil, melted
- 2 tablespoons cocoa powder

Directions:

1. In a blender, combine the nectarines with the sugar and the rest of the ingredients, pulse well, pour into a lined square pan, spread, bake in the oven at 375 degrees F

for 20 minutes, leave the mix aside to cool down a bit, cut into squares and serve.

Nutrition info per serving: 221calories, 3.1g protein, 17.2g carbohydrates, 17.8g fat, 3.4g fiber, 0g cholesterol, 162mg sodium, 282g potassium

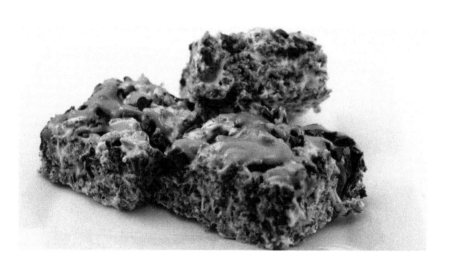

Grapes and Lime Compote

Preparation time: 10 minutes

Cooking time: 20 minutes

Servings: 4

Ingredients:

- 1 cup of green grapes
- Juice of ½ lime
- 2 tablespoons coconut sugar
- 1 and ½ cups of water
- 2 teaspoons cardamom powder

Directions:

1. Heat a pan with the water medium heat, add the grapes and the other ingredients, bring to a simmer, cook for 20 minutes, divide into bowls and serve.

Nutrition info per serving: 46calories, 0.5g protein, 12.4g carbohydrates, 0.2g fat, 1g fiber, 0g cholesterol, 3mg sodium, 75g potassium

Mandarin Cream

Preparation time: 10 minutes

Cooking time: 20 minutes

Servings: 4

Ingredients:

- 1 mandarin, peeled and chopped
- ½ pound plums, pitted and chopped
- 1 cup coconut cream
- Juice of 2 mandarins
- 2 tablespoons coconut sugar

Directions:

1. In a blender, combine the mandarin with the plums and the other ingredients, pulse well, divide into small ramekins, introduce in the oven, bake at 350 degrees F for 20 minutes, and serve cold.

Nutrition info per serving: 196calories, 1.7g protein, 18.1g carbohydrates, 14.5g fat, 1.6g fiber, 0g cholesterol, 26mg sodium, 281g potassium

Cherry Cream

Preparation time: 10 minutes

Cooking time: 0 minutes

Servings: 6

Ingredients:

- 1 pound cherries, pitted
- 1 cup strawberries, chopped
- ¼ cup of coconut sugar
- 2 cups coconut cream

Directions:

1. In a blender, combine the cherries with the other ingredients, pulse well, divide into bowls and serve cold.

Nutrition info per serving: 309calories, 2.3g protein, 35.4g carbohydrates, 19.2g fat, 2.7g fiber, 0g cholesterol, 26mg sodium, 327g potassium

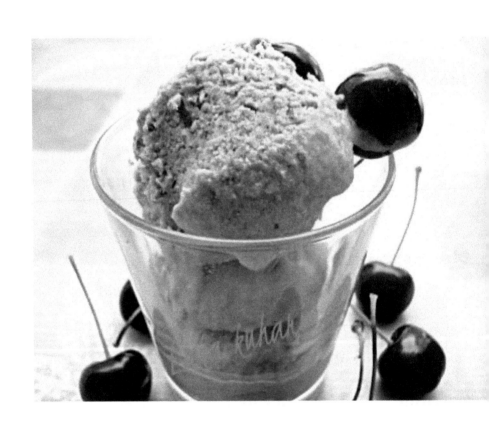

Walnuts Pudding

Preparation time: 5 minutes

Cooking time: 40 minutes

Servings: 4

Ingredients:

- 1 cup brown rice

- 3 cups almond milk

- 3 tablespoons coconut sugar

- ½ teaspoon cardamom powder

- ¼ cup walnuts, chopped

Directions:

1. In a pan, combine the rice with the milk and the other ingredients, stir, cook for 40 minutes over medium heat, divide into bowls and serve cold.

Nutrition info per serving: 666calories, 9.3g protein, 56.9g carbohydrates, 47.9g fat, 5.2g fiber, 0g cholesterol, 30mg sodium, 570g potassium

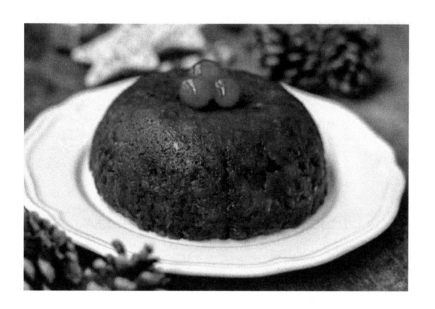

Fruity Bread

Preparation time: 10 minutes

Cooking time: 30 minutes

Servings: 4

Ingredients:

- 2 cups pears, cored and cubed
- 1 cup of coconut sugar
- 2 eggs, whisked
- 2 cups almond flour
- 1 tablespoon baking powder
- 1 tablespoon coconut oil, melted

Directions:

1. In a bowl, mix the pears with the sugar and the other ingredients, whisk, pour into a loaf pan, introduce in the oven, and bake at 350 degrees F for 30 minutes.
2. Slice and serve cold.

Nutrition info per serving: 371calories, 6.1g protein, 65.2g carbohydrates, 12.7g fat, 4.1g fiber, 82g cholesterol, 40mg sodium, 502g potassium

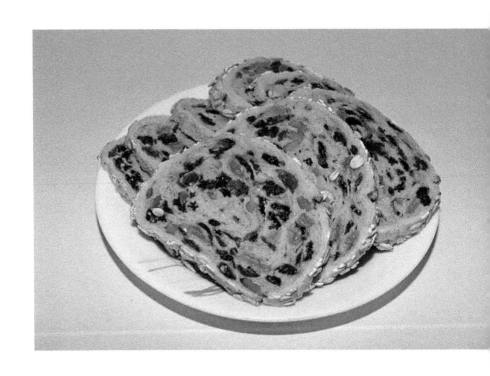

Vanilla Rice Pudding

Preparation time: 10 minutes

Cooking time: 25 minutes

Servings: 4

Ingredients:

- 1 tablespoon coconut oil, melted
- 1 cup brown rice
- 3 cups almond milk
- ½ cup cherries, pitted and halved
- 3 tablespoons coconut sugar
- 1 teaspoon cinnamon powder
- 1 teaspoon vanilla extract

Directions:

1. In a pan, combine the oil with the rice and the other ingredients, stir, bring to a simmer, cook for 25 minutes over medium heat, divide into bowls and serve cold.

Nutrition info per serving: 291calories, 4.1g protein, 54.7g carbohydrates, 5.6g fat, 0.7g fiber, 0g cholesterol, 109mg sodium, 64g potassium

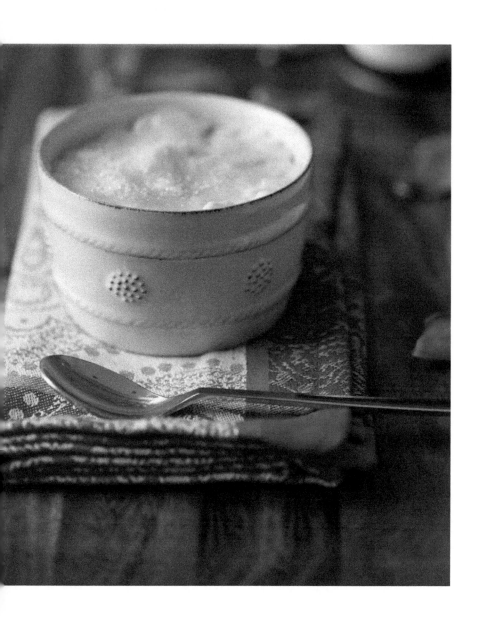

Lime Watermelon Compote

Preparation time: 5 minutes

Cooking time: 8 minutes

Servings: 4

Ingredients:

- Juice of 1 lime

- 1 teaspoon lime zest, grated

- 1 and ½ cup of coconut sugar

- 4 cups watermelon, peeled and cut into large chunks

- 1 and ½ cups of water

Directions:

1. In a pan, combine the watermelon with the lime zest, and the other ingredients, toss, bring to a simmer over medium heat, cook

for 8 minutes, divide into bowls and serve cold.

Nutrition info per serving: 386calories, 1g protein, 103.3g carbohydrates, 0.2g fat, 1.1g fiber, 0.2g cholesterol, 200mg sodium, 187g potassium

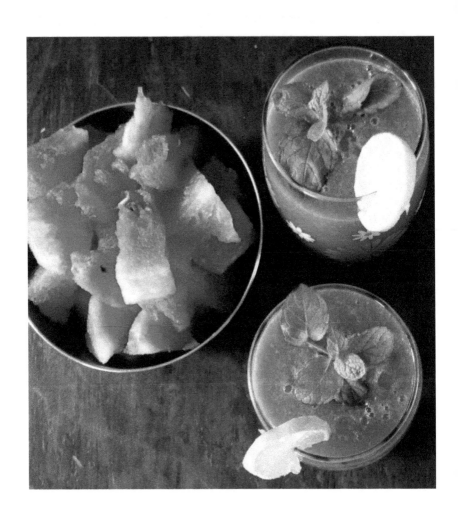

Ginger Chia Pudding

Preparation time: 1 hour

Cooking time: 0 minutes

Servings: 4

Ingredients:

- 2 cups almond milk
- ½ cup coconut cream
- 2 tablespoons coconut sugar
- 1 tablespoon ginger, grated
- ¼ cup chia seeds

Directions:

1. In a bowl, combine the milk with the cream and the other ingredients, whisk well, divide into small cups and keep them in the fridge for 1 hour before serving.

Nutrition info per serving: 188calories, 3.2g protein, 16.1g carbohydrates, 13.4g fat, 3.8g fiber, 1g cholesterol, 11mg sodium, 126g potassium

Lemon Cashew Cream

Preparation time: 2 hours

Cooking time: 0 minutes

Servings: 4

Ingredients:

- 1 cup cashews, chopped

- 2 tablespoons coconut oil, melted

- 1 cup coconut cream

- tablespoons lemon juice

- 1 tablespoon coconut sugar

Directions:

1. In a blender, combine the cashews with the coconut oil and the other ingredients, pulse well, divide into small cups and keep in the fridge for 2 hours before serving.

Nutrition info per serving: 404calories, 6.6g protein, 17.5g carbohydrates, 37g fat, 2.4g fiber, 0g cholesterol, 14mg sodium, 351g potassium

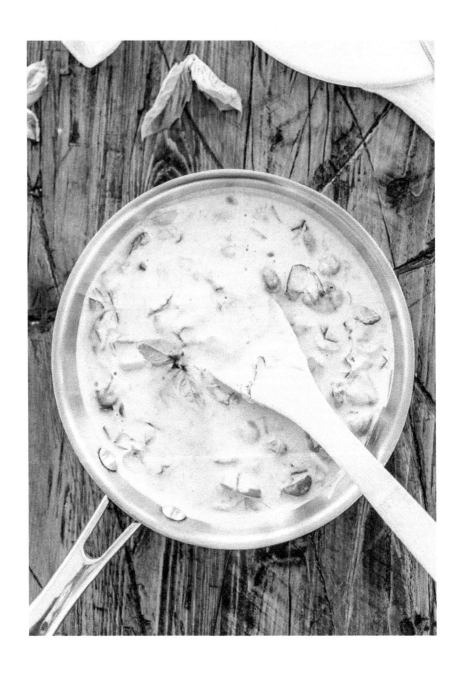

Coconut Hemp and Almond Cookies

Preparation time: 30 minutes

Cooking time: 0 minutes

Servings: 6

Ingredients:

- 1 cup almonds, soaked overnight and drained
- 2 tablespoons cocoa powder
- 1 tablespoon coconut sugar
- ½ cup hemp seeds
- ¼ cup coconut, shredded
- ½ cup of water

Directions:

1. In your food processor, combine the almonds with the cocoa powder and the other ingredients, pulse well, press this on

a lined baking sheet, keep in the fridge for 30 minutes, slice, and serve.

Nutrition info per serving: 185calories, 8g protein, 7.7g carbohydrates, 15g fat, 3.2g fiber, 0g cholesterol, 2mg sodium, 290g potassium

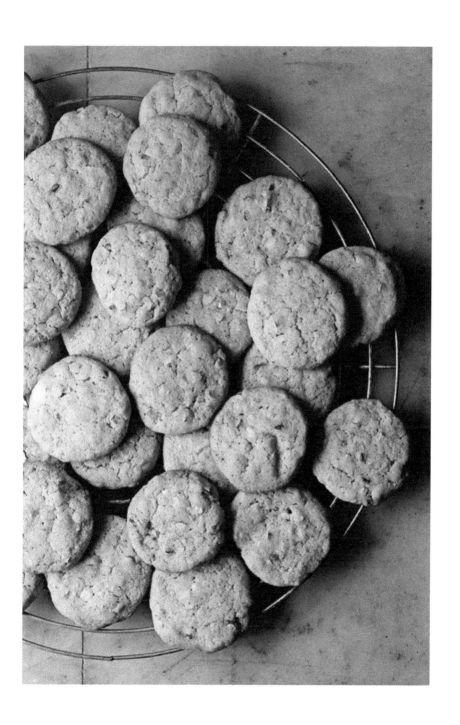

Coconut Pomegranate Bowls

Preparation time: 2 hours

Cooking time: 0 minutes

Servings: 4

Ingredients:

- ½ cup coconut cream
- 1 teaspoon vanilla extract
- 1 cup almonds, chopped
- 1 cup pomegranate seeds
- 1 tablespoon coconut sugar

Directions:

1. In a bowl, combine the almonds with the cream and the other ingredients, toss, divide into small bowls and serve.

Nutrition info per serving: 246calories, 6g protein, 15.9g carbohydrates, 19g fat, 3.9g fiber, 0g cholesterol, 5mg sodium, 255g potassium

Vanilla Chia Cream

Preparation time: 10 minutes

Cooking time: 0 minutes

Servings: 6

Ingredients:

- 2 cups coconut cream
- 2/3 cup coconut sugar
- 1 cup almond milk
- 3 tablespoons chia seeds, ground
- ½ teaspoon vanilla extract

Directions:

1. In a bowl, combine the cream with the chia seeds and the other ingredients, whisk well, divide into small bowls, leave aside for 10 minutes and serve.

Nutrition info per serving: 510calories, 5.3g protein, 54.7g carbohydrates, 33.6g fat, 7.5g fiber, 0g cholesterol, 143mg sodium, 374g potassium

Ginger Berries Bowls

Preparation time: 5 minutes

Cooking time: 0 minutes

Servings: 4

Ingredients:

- 1 cup blackberries

- 1 cup blueberries

- 1 tablespoon lime juice

- 1 cup strawberries, halved

- 1 tablespoon coconut sugar

- ½ teaspoon ginger powder

- ½ teaspoon vanilla extract

Directions:

1. In a bowl, combine the blackberries with the blueberries and the other ingredients, toss and serve.

Nutrition info per serving: 62calories, 1.1g protein, 15g carbohydrates, 0.4g fat, 3.6g fiber, 0g cholesterol, 2mg sodium, 148g potassium

Grapefruit and Coconut Cream

Preparation time: 10 minutes

Cooking time: 10 minutes

Servings: 4

Ingredients:

- 1 cup of coconut milk

- 2 tablespoons coconut sugar

- ½ cup coconut cream

- 1 teaspoon vanilla extract

- 4 grapefruits, peeled and roughly chopped

Directions:

1. In a pan, combine the milk with the grapefruits and the other ingredients, whisk, bring to a simmer and cook over medium heat for 10 minutes.

2. Blend using an immersion blender, divide into bowls and serve cold.

Nutrition info per serving: 204calories, 2.2g protein, 19.8g carbohydrates, 14.4g fat, 2.7g fiber, 0g cholesterol, 9mg sodium, 337g potassium

Walnuts Cream

Preparation time: 10 minutes

Cooking time: 0 minutes

Servings: 6

Ingredients:

- 3 cups non-fat milk

- 1 teaspoon nutmeg, ground

- 2 teaspoons vanilla extract

- 4 teaspoons coconut sugar

- 1 cup walnuts, chopped

Directions:

1. In a bowl, combine milk with the nutmeg and the other ingredients, whisk well, divide into small cups and serve cold.

Nutrition info per serving: 190calories, 9g protein, 11.1g carbohydrates, 12.4g fat, 1.5g fiber, 2g cholesterol, 66mg sodium, 302mg potassium

Coconut Avocado Cream

Preparation time: 1 hour and 10 minutes

Cooking time: 0 minutes

Servings: 4

Ingredients:

- 2 cups coconut cream

- 2 avocados, peeled, pitted and mashed

- 2 tablespoons coconut sugar

- 1 teaspoon vanilla extract

Directions:

1. In a blender, combine the cream with the avocados and the other ingredients, pulse well, divide into cups and keep in the fridge for 1 hour before serving.

Nutrition info per serving: 512calories, 4.7g protein, 22.9g carbohydrates, 48.2g fat, 9.4g fiber, 0g cholesterol, 41mg sodium, 805g potassium

Raspberries and Cream Cheese Mix

Preparation time: 10 minutes

Cooking time: 25 minutes

Servings: 4

Ingredients:

- 2 tablespoons almond flour

- 1 cup coconut cream

- 3 cups raspberries

- 1 cup of coconut sugar

- 8 ounces low-fat cream cheese

Directions:

1. In a bowl, the flour with the cream and the other ingredients, whisk, transfer to a round pan, cook at 360 degrees F for 25 minutes, divide into bowls and serve.

Nutrition info per serving: 644calories, 9.8g protein, 66.8g carbohydrates, 41.7g fat, 8.8g fiber, 62g cholesterol, 183mg sodium, 365g potassium

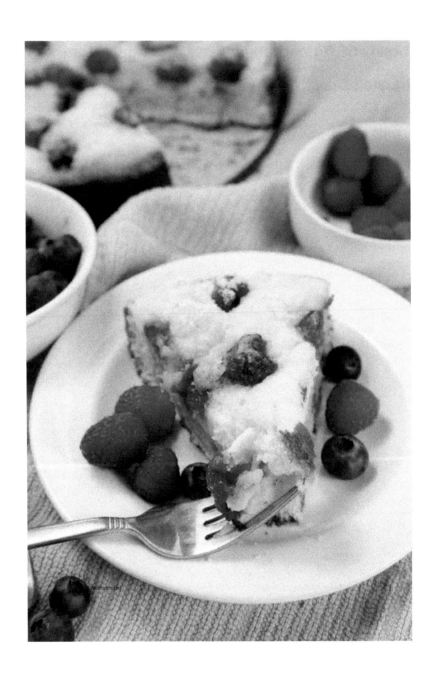

Watermelon and Apples Salad

Preparation time: 4 minutes

Cooking time: 0 minutes

Servings: 4

Ingredients:

- 1 cup watermelon, peeled and cubed

- 2 apples, cored and cubed

- 1 tablespoon coconut cream

- 2 bananas, cut into chunks

Directions:

1. In a bowl, combine the watermelon with the apples and the other ingredients, toss and serve.

Nutrition info per serving: 131calories, 1.3g protein, 31.9g carbohydrates, 1.3g fat, 4.5g fiber, 0g cholesterol, 3mg sodium, 383g potassium

Lime Pears Mix

Preparation time: 10 minutes

Cooking time: 10 minutes

Servings: 4

Ingredients:

- 2 teaspoons lime juice
- ½ cup coconut cream
- ½ cup coconut, shredded
- 4 pears, cored and cubed
- 4 tablespoons coconut sugar

Directions:

1. In a pan, combine the pears with the lime juice and the other ingredients, stir, bring to a simmer over medium heat and cook for 10 minutes.
2. Divide into bowls and serve cold.

Nutrition info per serving: 281calories, 1.8g protein, 50g carbohydrates, 10.8g fat, 8g fiber, 0g cholesterol, 42mg sodium, 357g potassium

Orange Compote

Preparation time: 10 minutes

Cooking time: 15 minutes

Servings: 4

Ingredients:

- 5 tablespoons coconut sugar
- 2 cups orange juice
- 4 apples, cored and cubed

Directions:

1. In a pot, combine apples with the sugar and the orange juice, toss, bring to a boil over medium heat, cook for 15 minutes, divide into bowls and serve cold.

Nutrition info per serving: 242calories, 1.5g protein, 62.5g carbohydrates, 0.7g fat, 5.7g fiber, 0g cholesterol, 44mg sodium, 487g potassium

Apricots Compote

Preparation time: 10 minutes

Cooking time: 15 minutes

Servings: 4

Ingredients:

- 2 cups apricots, halved
- 2 cups of water
- 2 tablespoons coconut sugar
- 2 tablespoons lemon juice

Directions:

1. In a pot, combine the apricots with the water and the other ingredients, toss, cook over medium heat for 15 minutes, divide into bowls and serve.

Nutrition info per serving: 63calories, 1.1g protein, 14.7g carbohydrates, 0.6g fat, 1.5g fiber, 0g cholesterol, 6mg sodium, 211g potassium

Vanilla Cantaloupe Bowls

Preparation time: 10 minutes

Cooking time: 10 minutes

Servings: 4

Ingredients:

- 2 cups cantaloupe, peeled and roughly cubed
- 4 tablespoons coconut sugar
- 2 teaspoons vanilla extract
- 2 teaspoons lemon juice

Directions:

1. In a small pan, combine the cantaloupe with the sugar and the other ingredients, toss, heat up over medium heat, cook for about 10 minutes, divide into bowls and serve cold.

Nutrition info per serving: 89calories, 0.7g protein, 21.7g carbohydrates, 0.2g fat, 0.7g fiber, 0g cholesterol, 46mg sodium, 215g potassium

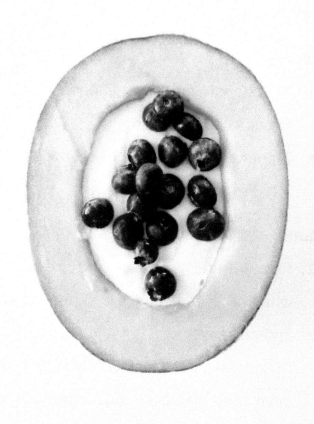

Rhubarb Cream

Preparation time: 10 minutes

Cooking time: 14 minutes

Servings: 4

Ingredients:

- 1/3 cup low-fat cream cheese
- ½ cup coconut cream
- 2-pound rhubarb, roughly chopped
- 3 tablespoons coconut sugar

Directions:

1. In a blender, combine the cream cheese with the cream and the other ingredients and pulse well.
2. Divide into small cups, introduce in the oven, and bake at 350 degrees F for 14 minutes.
3. Serve cold.

Nutrition info per serving: 218calories, 4.2g protein, 21.5g carbohydrates, 14.3g fat, 4.7g fiber, 21g cholesterol, 71mg sodium, 755g potassium

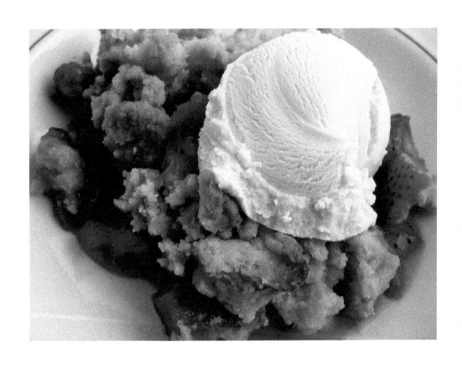

Mint Pineapple Mix

Preparation time: 10 minutes

Cooking time: 0 minutes

Servings: 4

Ingredients:

- 3 cups pineapple, peeled and cubed

- 1 teaspoon chia seeds

- 1 cup coconut cream

- 1 teaspoon vanilla extract

- 1 tablespoon mint, chopped

Directions:

1. In a bowl, combine the pineapple with the cream and the other ingredients, toss, divide into smaller bowls and keep in the fridge for 10 minutes before serving.

Nutrition info per serving: 215calories, 2.5g protein, 20.8g carbohydrates, 15.2g fat, 4g fiber, 0g cholesterol, 11mg sodium, 311g potassium

Berry Compote

Preparation time: 10 minutes

Cooking time: 10 minutes

Servings: 4

Ingredients:

- 2 tablespoons lemon juice

- 1 cup of water

- 3 tablespoons coconut sugar

- 12 ounces blueberries

Directions:

1. In a pan, combine the blueberries with the sugar and the other ingredients, bring to a gentle simmer and cook over medium heat for 10 minutes.
2. Divide into bowls and serve.

Nutrition info per serving: 87calories, 0.7g protein, 21.5g carbohydrates, 0.4g fat, 2.1g fiber, 0g cholesterol, 4mg sodium, 76g potassium

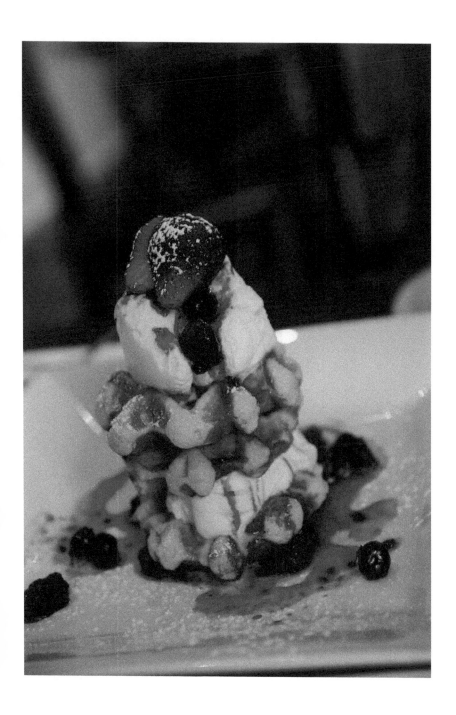

Lime Coconut Pudding

Preparation time: 10 minutes

Cooking time: 15 minutes

Servings: 4

Ingredients:

- 2 cups coconut cream

- Juice of 1 lime

- Zest of 1 lime, grated

- 3 tablespoons coconut oil, melted

- 1 egg, whisked

- 1 teaspoon baking powder

Directions:

1. In a bowl, combine the cream with the lime juice and the other ingredients and whisk well.

2. Divide into small ramekins, introduce in the oven, and bake at 360 degrees F for 15 minutes.
3. Serve the pudding cold.

Nutrition info per serving: 386calories, 4.4g protein, 9.1g carbohydrates, 39.9g fat, 3.2g fiber, 41g cholesterol, 35mg sodium, 475g potassium

Almond Cream

Preparation time: 10 minutes

Cooking time: 0 minutes

Servings: 4

Ingredients:

- 3 cups coconut cream
- 2 peaches, stones removed and chopped
- 1 teaspoon vanilla extract
- ½ cup almonds, chopped

Directions:

1. In a blender, combine the cream and the other ingredients, pulse well, divide into small bowls and serve cold.

Nutrition info per serving: 515calories, 7.3g protein, 19.7g carbohydrates, 49.1g fat, 6.6g fiber, 0g cholesterol, 27mg sodium, 705g potassium

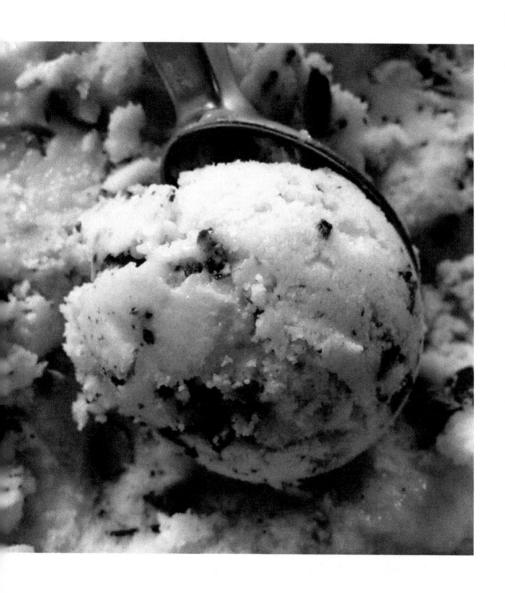

Sweet Plums Mix

Preparation time: 10 minutes

Cooking time: 15 minutes

Servings: 4

Ingredients:

- 1 pound plums, stones removed and halved
- 2 tablespoons coconut sugar
- ½ teaspoon cinnamon powder
- 1 cup of water

Directions:

1. In a pan, combine the plums with the sugar and the other ingredients, bring to a simmer and cook over medium heat for 15 minutes.
2. Divide into bowls and serve cold.

Nutrition info per serving: 30calories, 0.1g protein, 8g carbohydrates, 0.1g fat, 0.2g fiber, 0g cholesterol, 2mg sodium, 27g potassium

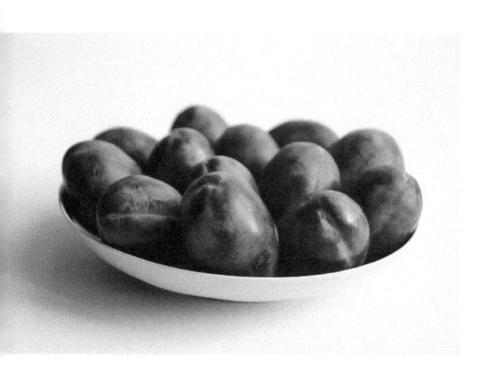

Chia Apples Mix

Preparation time: 10 minutes

Cooking time: 10 minutes

Servings: 4

Ingredients:

- 2 cups apples, cored and cut into wedges
- 2 tablespoons chia seeds
- 1 teaspoon vanilla extract
- 2 cups naturally unsweetened apple juice

Directions:

1. In a small pot, combine the apples with the chia seeds and the other ingredients, toss, cook over medium heat for 10 minutes, divide into bowls and serve cold.

Nutrition info per serving: 155calories, 1.5g protein, 33.5g carbohydrates, 2.4g fat, 5.1g fiber, 0g cholesterol, 15mg sodium, 240g potassiumx

Rice Pudding

Preparation time: 10 minutes

Cooking time: 25 minutes

Servings: 4

Ingredients:

- 6 cups of water
- 1 cup of coconut sugar
- 2 cups black rice
- 2 pears, cored and cubed
- 2 teaspoons cinnamon powder

Directions:

1. Put the water in a pan, heat it over medium-high heat, add the rice, sugar and the other ingredients, stir, bring to a simmer, reduce heat to medium and cook for 25 minutes.
2. Divide into bowls and serve cold.

Nutrition info per serving: 340calories, 2.4g protein, 85.3g carbohydrates, 0.8g fat, 3.9g fiber, 0g cholesterol, 12mg sodium, 191g potassium

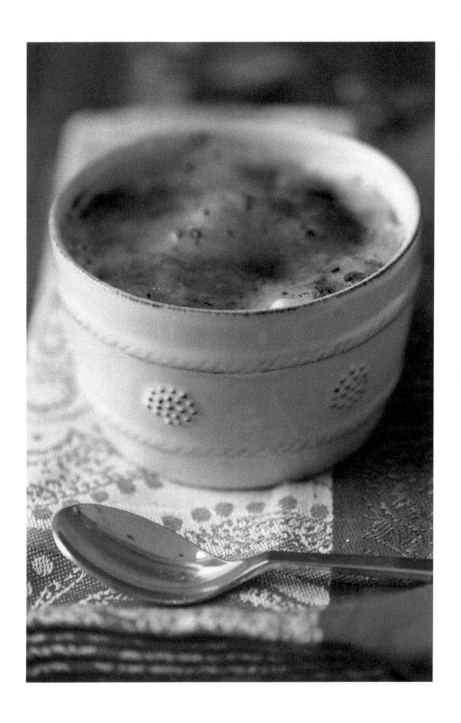

Rhubarb Compote

Preparation time: 10 minutes

Cooking time: 15 minutes

Servings: 4

Ingredients:

- 2 cups rhubarb, roughly chopped
- 3 tablespoons coconut sugar
- 1 teaspoon almond extract
- 2 cups of water

Directions:

1. In a pot, combine the rhubarb with the other ingredients, toss, bring to a boil over medium heat, cook for 15 minutes, divide into bowls and serve cold.

Nutrition info per serving: 52calories, 0.6g protein, 11.9g carbohydrates, 0.1g fat, 1.1g fiber, 0g cholesterol, 6mg sodium, 178g potassium

Coconut Rhubarb Cream

Preparation time: 1 hour

Cooking time: 10 minutes

Servings: 4

Ingredients:

- 2 cups coconut cream
- 1 cup rhubarb, chopped
- 3 eggs, whisked
- 3 tablespoons coconut sugar
- 1 tablespoon lime juice

Directions:

1. In a small pan, combine the cream with the rhubarb and the other ingredients, whisk well, simmer over medium heat for 10 minutes, blend using an immersion blender, divide into bowls and keep in the fridge for 1 hour before serving.

Nutrition info per serving: 363calories, 7.2g protein, 17.3g carbohydrates, 32g fat, 3.2g fiber, 123g cholesterol, 65mg sodium, 448g potassium

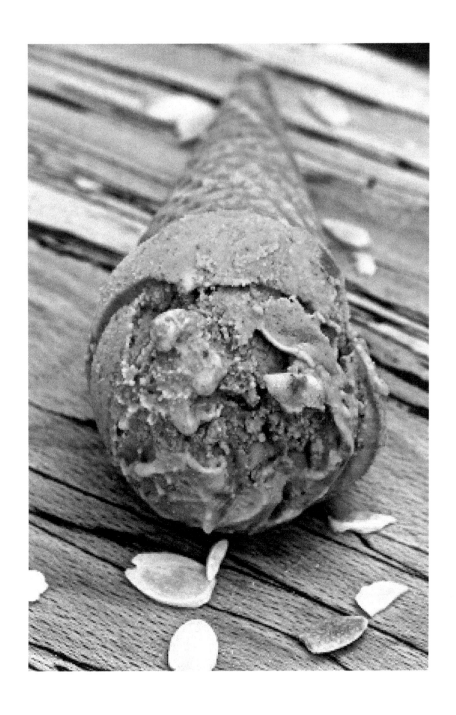

Minty Fruit Salad

Preparation time: 5 minutes

Cooking time: 0 minutes

Servings: 4

Ingredients:

- 2 cups blueberries
- 3 tablespoons mint, chopped
- 1 pear, cored and cubed
- 1 apple, cored, cubed
- 1 tablespoon coconut sugar

Directions:

1. In a bowl, combine the blueberries with the mint and the other ingredients, toss, and serve cold.

Nutrition info per serving: 104calories, 1g protein, 26.9g carbohydrates, 0.4g fat, 4.5g fiber, 123g cholesterol, 3mg sodium, 175g potassium

Dates Cream

Preparation time: 5 minutes

Cooking time: 0 minutes

Servings: 4

Ingredients:

- 1 cup almond milk

- 1 banana, peeled and sliced

- 1 teaspoon vanilla extract

- ½ cup coconut cream

- 1 cup dates, chopped

Directions:

1. In a blender, combine the dates with the banana and the other ingredients, pulse well, divide into small cups and serve cold.

Nutrition info per serving: 119calories, 1.3g protein, 12.1g carbohydrates, 7.9g fat, 1.6g fiber, 0g cholesterol, 40mg sodium, 200g potassiumx

Almond Plum Muffins

Preparation time: 10 minutes

Cooking time: 25 minutes

Servings: 12

Ingredients:

- 3 tablespoons coconut oil, melted
- ½ cup almond milk
- 4 eggs, whisked
- 1 teaspoon vanilla extract
- 1 cup almond flour
- 2 teaspoons cinnamon powder
- ½ teaspoon baking powder
- 1 cup plums, pitted and chopped

Directions:

1. In a bowl, combine the coconut oil with the almond milk and the other ingredients and whisk well.

2. Divide into a muffin pan, introduce in the oven at 350 degrees F and bake for 25 minutes.
3. Serve the muffins cold.

Nutrition info per serving: 137calories, 2.1g protein, 3.1g carbohydrates, 12.3g fat, 1.3g fiber, 55g cholesterol, 22mg sodium, 76g potassium

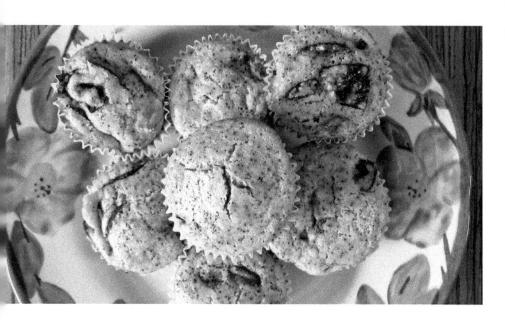

Coconut Plums Bowls

Preparation time: 10 minutes

Cooking time: 20 minutes

Servings: 4

Ingredients:

- ½ pound plums, pitted and halved

- 2 tablespoons coconut sugar

- 4 tablespoons raisins

- 1 teaspoon vanilla extract

- 1 cup coconut cream

Directions:

1. In a pan, combine the plums with the sugar and the other ingredients, bring to a simmer and cook over medium heat for 20 minutes.
2. Divide into bowls and serve.

Nutrition info per serving: 194calories, 1.7g protein, 17.6g carbohydrates, 14.4g fat, 1.8g fiber, 0g cholesterol, 10mg sodium, 240g potassium

Seed Energy Bars

Preparation time: 10 minutes

Cooking time: 20 minutes

Servings: 6

Ingredients:

- 1 cup coconut flour

- ½ teaspoon baking soda

- 1 tablespoon flax seed

- 3 tablespoons almond milk

- 1 cup sunflower seeds

- 2 tablespoons coconut oil, melted

- 1 teaspoon vanilla extract

Directions:

1. In a bowl, mix the flour with the baking soda and the other ingredients, stir well, spread on a baking sheet, press well, bake

in the oven at 350 degrees F for 20 minutes, leave aside to cool down, cut into bars and serve.

Nutrition info per serving: 189calories, 4.7g protein, 13g carbohydrates, 13.3g fat, 7.8g fiber, 0g cholesterol, 146mg sodium, 80g potassium

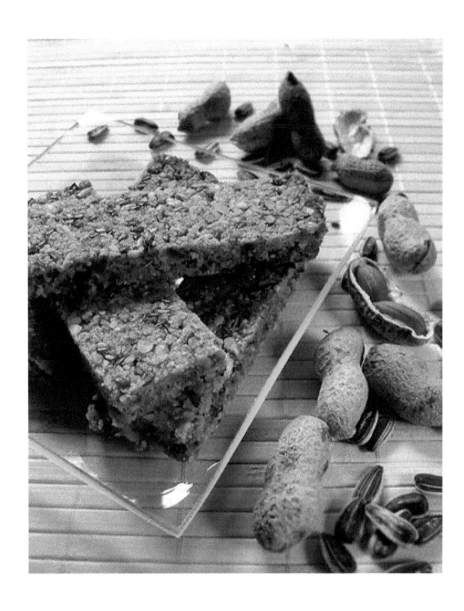

Blackberries Salad

Preparation time: 10 minutes

Cooking time: 0 minutes

Servings: 4

Ingredients:

- 1 cup cashews
- 2 cups blackberries
- ¾ cup coconut cream
- 1 teaspoon vanilla extract
- 1 tablespoon coconut sugar

Directions:

1. In a bowl, combine the cashews with the berries and the other ingredients, toss, divide into small bowls and serve.

Nutrition info per serving: 348calories, 7.3g protein, 24.5g carbohydrates, 27g fat, 5.8g fiber, 0g cholesterol, 21mg sodium, 430g potassium

Orange Salad

Preparation time: 4 minutes

Cooking time: 8 minutes

Servings: 4

Ingredients:

- 4 oranges, peeled and cut into segments
- 2 tangerines, peeled and cut into segments
- Juice of 1 lime
- 2 tablespoons coconut sugar
- 1 cup of water

Directions:

1. In a pan, combine the oranges with the tangerines and the other ingredients, bring to a simmer and cook over medium heat for 8 minutes.
2. Divide into bowls and serve cold.

Nutrition info per serving: 158calories, 2.6g protein, 37.6g carbohydrates, 0.4g fat, 5.5g fiber, 0g cholesterol, 23mg sodium, 409g potassium

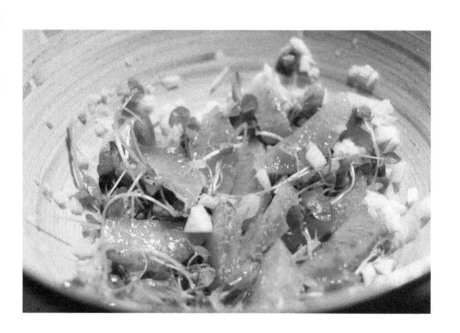